The Type 2 Diabetes Cure

How To Naturally Prevent & Reverse Type 2 Diabetes

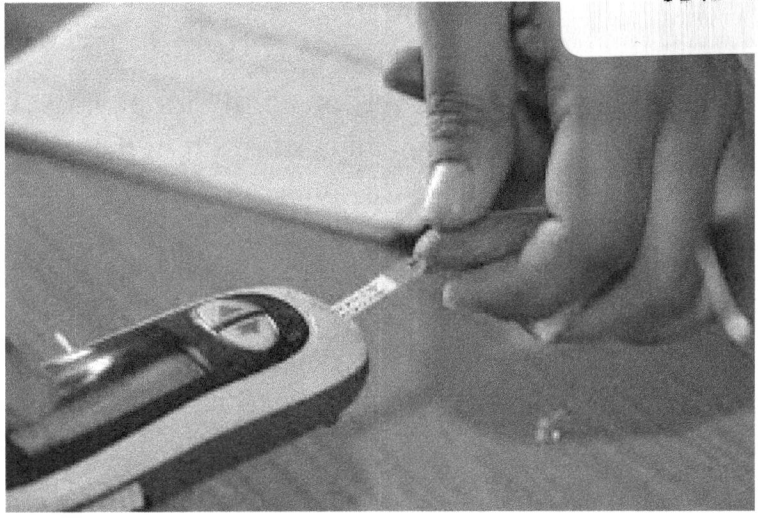

Disclaimer

This book is intended to be a general guide, to raise awareness, and to help people make informed decisions in the context of their own personal circumstance.

As everybody's circumstances are different, so are the remedies you should seek. While many of the recommendations in this book can be applied by almost anybody regardless of their conditions, they are not intended to and should not be relied upon to replace personal medical advice.

The author accepts no responsibility for any loss or injury, be it personal or financial, as a result of the use or misuse of the information in this book.

If you have any doubts or concerns after reading this book, please speak to a doctor or other qualified person before taking any actions.

From The Author

Thank you for taking the time to read this book. As an author, I understand the importance of creating books which my readers will find both enjoyable and informative. If you have the time and feel generous, please don't hesitate to leave an honest review of this book.........Dr Brad Turner

Contents

Introduction

According to the World Health Organization (WHO, 2013), there are 347 million people suffering from diabetes all over the world. WHO also projects that diabetes will be the seventh leading cause of death when the year 2030 arrives. With this in mind, can it still be prevented or reversed? This would be one of the most vital questions that someone who has been diagnosed with diabetes would ask.

Diabetes is generally referred as a chronic disease that has something to do with the inability of either the pancreas to produce enough insulin or of the body to effectively use the insulin that it produces. Insulin is a vital hormone, which regulates the blood sugar. Hyperglycemia, also known as high blood sugar, is the common effect of uncontrolled diabetes. Over time, this condition leads to serious, and even fatal, damage to various systems of the body, most especially the blood vessels and nerves.

There are different kinds of diabetes. Three (3) of the most common types are Type 1, Type 2 and Gestational Diabetes.

Type 1, on the one hand, is about insulin production deficiency, which is common among young people. Among its reported symptoms are polyuria, polydipsia, constant hunger, weight loss, visual changes and even fatigue.

Type 2, on the other hand, is about the ineffective use of insulin of the body. This will be the focus of this paper, since 90% of people around the world with diabetes have this type, according to WHO (1999). Moreover, the third common type is Gestational Diabetes, which is special because it occurs during pregnancy.

However, this condition may still stick to both the mother and the baby even after conception, most especially when not addressed appropriately.

In terms of prevention, there are definitely some effective ways in order to prevent diabetes from fully developing. These ways should be done upon the earliest onset of symptoms. On the other hand, in terms of reversibility, some would say that it is quite debatable, but experts also claim that it is still possible.

Chapter 1

What Is Type 2 Diabetes?

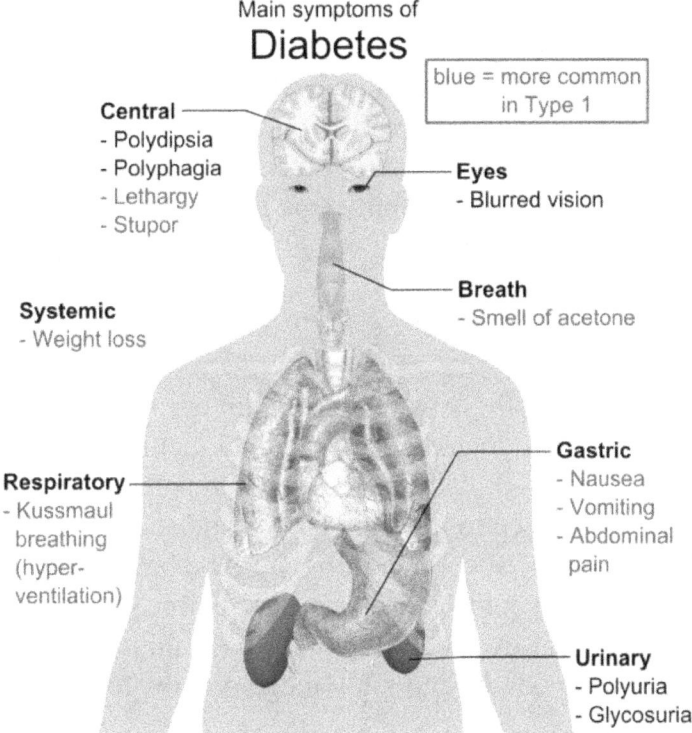

Main symptoms of
Diabetes

blue = more common in Type 1

Central
- Polydipsia
- Polyphagia
- Lethargy
- Stupor

Eyes
- Blurred vision

Breath
- Smell of acetone

Systemic
- Weight loss

Respiratory
- Kussmaul breathing (hyper-ventilation)

Gastric
- Nausea
- Vomiting
- Abdominal pain

Urinary
- Polyuria
- Glycosuria

Above: Shows the general symptoms of diabetes

Type 2 diabetes was usually called non-insulin dependent or adult-onset diabetes. The former name is because of its nature while the latter is because it was more commonly diagnosed in adult patients before. However, this may also occur at any age. In terms of its signs or symptoms, most of the people with Type 2 diabetes are not aware of their condition until they undergo blood or urine glucose tests. These tests are usually part of pre-employment medical requirements.

Moreover, though not always the case, Type 2 diabetes is often associated with overweight or obese people.

When it comes to the management of this condition, high glucose levels can be controlled. There is even a high chance of decreasing it by engaging in more physical activities and having a balanced healthy diet. In having a healthy diet, understanding blood sugar levels would be very vital. Hence, you need to know how to read it since this will tell you if your sugar level is high, normal, or low. This is especially true if you have already been diagnosed with this condition.

Understanding Blood Sugar Levels

There are two (2) options when checking your blood sugar level. One is to go to your doctor or to a medical facility to have your glucose level checked. Alternatively, you can also check it on your own. If you need to monitor your blood sugar level more often, then using the second option would be better than the hassle of going to your doctor every single time. However, checking it on your own will require two (2) things, which are investment in the device and knowledge on how to do it on your own.

It is a good thing that there is already do-it-yourself equipment that lets you do this on your own. Once you have that, the only thing you need to know is the normal range.

According to the National Institute of Clinical Excellence (NICE) (Diabetes Digital Media, n.d.), normal ranges of blood sugar level before and after meals are as follows:

Table 1. Pre and Post Prandial Target Glucose Levels

Target Levels by Type	Before meals (pre prandial)	2 hours after meals (post prandial)
Non-diabetic	4.0 to 5.9 mmol/L	under 7.8 mmol/L
Type 2 diabetes	4 to 7 mmol/L	under 8.5 mmol/L
Type 1 diabetes	4 to 7 mmol/L	under 9 mmol/L
Children w/ type 1 diabetes	4 to 8 mmol/L	under 10 mmol/L

However, you need to take note that these ranges are just guides and are not absolute or universally applicable. There are various factors that may affect and dictate the normal range for a particular person with any kind of diabetes. These factors usually include age, gender, and even medical history. Hence, it would be best to consult your doctor first in order to determine the normal range of blood sugar level, considering your condition.

Aside from the normal range, the regularity of monitoring is also essential. Like the specific range that would be applicable to a particular person, the frequency of monitoring varies as well. Some factors that may determine how frequently you should monitor it include the variance of your current blood sugar level from the normal range, as well as specific conditions (e.g. weight, obesity, hypertension, etc.) and the like.

There are some cases when a person with Type 2 diabetes needs to monitor his or her blood sugar level before and after every meal. This means that monitoring should be done at least six times a day. However, there are also some cases when the monitoring only needs to be done once a day or even weekly.

Such frequency is usually advised on patients that engage in healthy eating and exercise.

Chapter 2

The Importance Of Proper Nutrition On Diabetes

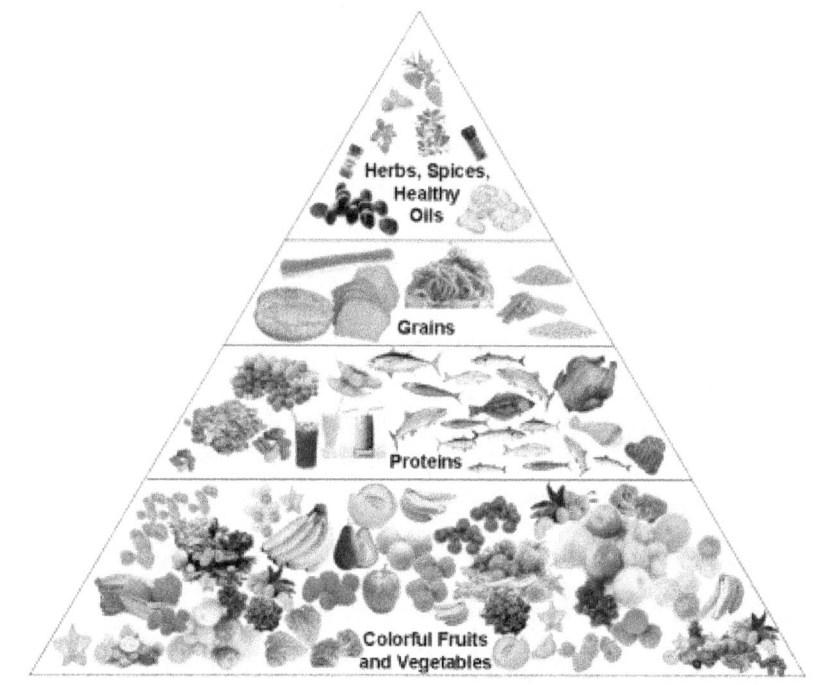

Above: The nutritional pyramid shows the food groups of which you should eat more

With Type 2 diabetes, most people think that people with this condition need to have a special diet and eating habits. Sadly, the mindset is more inclined toward eating less. However, it has to be clarified that healthy eating is not tantamount or equivalent to eating less. Rather, healthy eating should be about having proper nutrition.

In general, healthy diet maintains and improves one's general health. On the other hand, having a balanced diet is about taking the right amount and kind of food and drinks that will supply the necessary nutrition and energy to a person. Crash dieting is not healthy because it abruptly shifts the pattern of eating of a person. Whereas in a balanced healthy diet, proportion and types of food are considered.

For diabetic people, their diet should be in conjunction with their eating habits and actual condition. What makes things special in a healthy diet for diabetic people is that it specifically deals with sugar intake regulation. To reiterate, it is just to regulate rather than to eradicate sugar intake. This is because our bodies still need sugar and associated nutrients in order to make our body cells, tissues and organs function properly.

In this regard, there are some myths and misconceptions that need to be deconstructed when talking about proper nutrition and healthy diet for people with Type 2 diabetes.

Myth 1: Avoiding sugar
As stated above, it is not true that people with this condition need to avoid sugar at all costs. As a matter of fact, everyone needs it. However, for diabetic people, it just needs to be regulated. What this means is that you do not have to exclude desserts from your menu at all.

Myth 2: Choosing a high-protein diet
Too much protein may lead to insulin resistance, which will consequently result in diabetes. Instead, a person's diet should also contain a balanced combination of carbohydrates and fats, aside from protein. These are all needed in order to make the body function well.

Myth 3: It is a must to cut down your carbs

Some people think that cutting down carbs from the meal plan is a must. However, while many kinds of food with carbohydrates increase blood sugar level, there are good kinds of carbohydrates that you can serve at your table in the right size. The list may include whole grain carbs that are also rich in fibre, which helps your glucose level even out.

Myth 4: People with Type 2 diabetes need special meals

While this is partly true, it should be noted that it is not entirely and absolutely true as well. This is because it does not mean that you can no longer eat the types of food that other people eat just because you have Type 2 diabetes. Rather, the key here is moderation and making smart choices. There are some alternatives of a specific kind of food that you can eat. This will be explained in Chapter 4, while the index that will help you choose the right kind of food to buy will be discussed in the next chapter.

Chapter 3

A Diabetic Eating Plan

One of the most useful tools that will help a person with diabetes have a good diet plan is the Glycemic Index. GI is a tool that is designed to know the rate that a certain food turns to sugar in your body or system. This indicates which meals are categorized as slow-release and which are not. In other words, it gives an estimate of how much a gram of carbohydrate, for instance, in the food will raise the glucose level of the consumer. A food with high GI means that it will spike the blood sugar level more rapidly. The table below provides a simple guide to better understand GI:

Table 2. Meaning of Glycemic Index (GI)

Low GI (<55)	**Sugars are broken down slowly (Best choice)**
Moderate GI (56-69)	Sugars are broken down moderately (Limit intake)
High GI (>70)	Sugars are broken down quickly (Avoid)

Generally, meals with low GI are recommended due to the following reasons:

- It will help you prevent fluctuations of blood sugar levels.
- It will make you feel fuller for a longer period, which will consequently avoid cravings.
- It will consequently help you manage weight better.
- It helps in managing blood fats.
- It leads to a lower insulin level.

There is also a newer term, the glycemic load, which takes into account the amount of carbohydrates in the food. The load provides a more precise idea of the impact of a certain food on the blood sugar level.

There are online tools that help people determine the GI and load through food charts. However, instead of relying on those, Michael Moore developed three (3) broad classifications of food, namely:

1. **Fire** – meals under this classification have high GI, but low fibre and protein. This kind of food must be eaten less often. Fire food includes "white food" like white rice, pasta, bread, potatoes and baked goods; as well as sweets, chips and various processed food.
2. **Water** – this refers to free food, which you can eat as much as you want. Under this class are vegetables and fruits. However, fruit juices, dried fruits and even canned fruits will spike your blood sugar fast. Therefore, they are not considered water food.
3. **Coal** – meals under this classification have low GI, and are high in fibre and protein. These include nuts, seeds, lean meats, whole grains, beans, as well as seafood and alternatives of "white food" indicated below.

Table 3. Food alternatives

Less preferred	Better alternatives
White rice	Brown or wild rice
White potatoes (e.g. mashed potatoes or fries)	Sweet potatoes Winter Squash Cauliflower mash Yams
Ordinary pasta	Whole-wheat pasta
White bread	Whole-wheat or –grain bread
Sugary cereals	High-fibre cereals (e.g. Raisin Bran)
Instant oatmeal	Rolled oats Steel-cut oats
Cornflakes	Bran flakes
Corn	Leafy greens Peas

However, it should be noted that abruptly switching from high to low GI meals may be counterproductive, rather than helpful. With that, you might want to consider the following tips in switching:

- Include at least one food low in GI in each of your meals or snacks.
- Use vinegar or lemon juice for dressings and sauces since the acidity lowers the score of a food with high GI.
- Do not overcook carbohydrate-rich food because doing so will lead to an increase in its GI.
- Include a little protein in your meals and snacks.
- Take some non-starchy vegetables or even salads.

Chapter 4

Affordable Ways To Eat Healthy

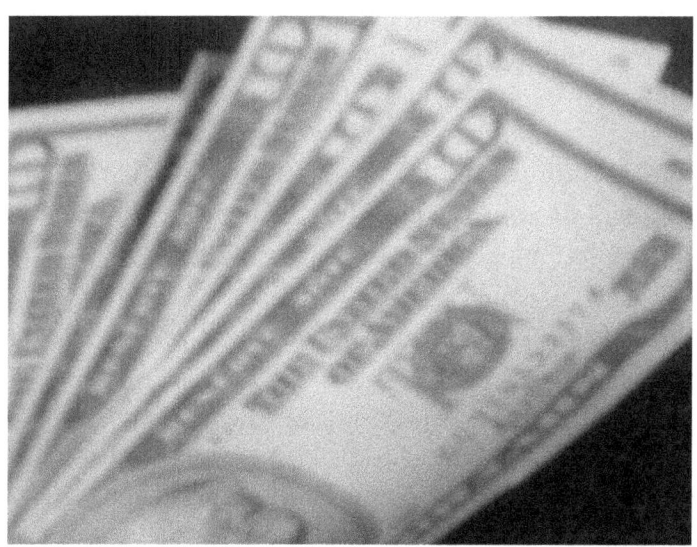

Now, one of the many trade offs of having a healthy diet is the cost. Well, this is because healthy food and meals tend to be more expensive than the junk ones. For instance, organic food is healthier, but more expensive than commercially-produced or even genetically-modified organisms (GMOs). This could be because organic food is not mass produced. However, this is not the only way to be healthy. There are, in fact, various tips and alternatives that you can explore in order to have an affordable healthy life.

Before getting to the tips and alternatives, it is crucial to know some guidelines first. These could be general or specific in nature, which include:

1. Changing the kind of food you eat

This is about changing both the kind of food you are eating and the manner in which you are eating them. The kinds of food that you should eat were partly discussed above while the manner refers to portion and frequency. In the previous chapter, the myth was debunked that eating less often is necessary. As a matter of fact, it is recommended to eat around six meals a day, but with moderate portions each meal. Aside from that, you should be particular on the contents of your meal too. The nutrition should be well distributed and balanced.

2. Choosing the right type of carbohydrates

The University of Maryland Medical Center (UMMC, n.d.) said that when food rich in carbohydrates is digested, it turns into a type of sugar, called blood glucose. However, it is still an essential component of anyone's diet. As stated also in the previous chapter, choosing the right type of carbohydrate is the right choice instead of eradicating carbs from your diet.

Usually, carbohydrates are found in foods like milk, fruits, yogurt, juices, rice, grain products, pasta, cereals, bread, bagels, rolls, crackers, dried beans, as well as potatoes and many more. Aside from those, common sweets are rich in carbohydrates too. These include honey, syrups, cookies, pastries, sodas and candies. However, there are alternatives to these kinds of food, aside from decreasing the amount of sugar.

3. *Food distribution*

As reiterated several times above, dieting is not primarily about reducing the frequency of eating. Rather, it is about distributing food quantity. You can have three full main meals in a day and another three snacks. However, moderation should still prevail.

4. *Reasonable portions*

In relation to the previous guide, the quality of the serving size is also important. The table above will help you choose the kinds of food that would be helpful to your diet, while not depriving you of the things that you want.

5. *Fruits are not always healthy*

Some people think that eating fruit is equivalent to being healthy. Well, it depends on the kind of fruits you are eating. There are fruits that are extremely high in sugar and GI. Of course, you should avoid those. You should beware of preserved and canned fruits, as well as powdered and any artificially produced or manufactured fruits. The quantity is a factor too. The recommended serving size is just a half of a cup. In this regard, "all natural" fruit extracts should be avoided too. This is because they are usually concentrated.

6. *Never skip meals*

Skipping meals is counterproductive, rather than helpful. It is true that glucose levels tend to be higher during mornings due to hormonal fluctuations. However, this is not a license to skip breakfast. With that, the specific kind of food for breakfast should be picked properly. For instance, you should avoid cereals, fruits and milk since they are quite difficult to tolerate.

7. *Limit, don't remove, sweets from your meals*

As deconstructed in the myths above, it is not true that you will never taste sweets again. Rather than removing them from your meals, you just need to be smart in picking the right kinds of sweets that you will eat. Of course, conventional sweets should be avoided as much as possible. The list includes cookies, cakes, candies and other food with excessive amounts of sugar. The reason behind this is that, aside from being rich in carbohydrates, these are also filled with fats, but little nutrition.

Sugar alcohols should be avoided too like mannitol, maltitol, sorbital, xylitol, isomalt and hydrogenated starch hydrolysate. Alternatively, there are artificial sweeteners that can be put on the food. These include aspartame (Equal, NutraSweet and Natra Taste), Acesulfame K (Sunnett) and Sucralose (Splenda).

Creating a Diet Plan (Some Tips and Alternative)

The following tips will guide diabetic people in creating their own diet plan.

Tip #1: Choose food with high fibre and slow-release carbohydrates

Experts say that carbohydrates have a great impact on increasing one's blood sugar. However, this does not mean that one should always avoid food rich in it. The trick here is to be smart in choosing the right kind of carbs.

As a general rule, it is ideal to limit one's intake of highly refined types of carbohydrates. These include, but are not limited to the following:

- White bread
- Pasta
- Rice
- Soda
- Candy
- Snack/junk food

Instead, a diabetic person should eat high-fibre complex types of carbohydrates. These are also called slow-release types of carbs, which help keep one's blood sugar level manageable because of their slow-digestion property. This will then prevent the body from producing so much insulin. Food with this kind of carbohydrate offers lasting energy that will make the consumer feel full longer. Some of these are indicated in Table 3 above.

Looking into the items in Table 3, it will be noticed that the bias of healthy and balanced diet plan for people with Type 2 diabetes is towards taking low-glycemic food. To be more specific about the kinds of food that diabetic people can eat, David Ludwig and Suzanne Rostler (2007) featured the following principles in "Ending the Food Fight:"

Table 4. "Ending the Food Fight" Principles

	Principle	Examples
1	Eat non-starchy food, specifically vegetables, beans and fruits	Apples, pears, peaches, berries, bananas, mangoes and papayas.
2	Eat least-processed grains	Whole-kernel bread, whole barley, millet, brown rice, wheat berries and traditionally processed stone-ground bread, natural granola and muesli cereals.
3	Eat less refined grain products	White potatoes, white breads, pasta and small side dishes.
4	Eat less concentrated sweets	Especially those with high caloric contents, though with low GI. Sugar-sweetened drinks are must-avoid here.
5	Eat healthy protein	Beans, fish and skinless chicken.
6	Pick healthful fats	Olive oil, almonds, pecans, almonds and avocados. Saturated, hydrogenated and trans fats should be avoided.
7	Eat regularly and never skip meals	3 full meals, 3 snacks in regulated sizes
8	Eat slowly and stop when full	

Tip #2: Be "sweet-smart"

As stated above, diabetic meals are not about eliminating sugar. Well, in fact, diabetic people can still enjoy a small quantity of their favorite desserts, but only in moderation. Discipline, conviction and lifestyle change would be vital here. This part will provide some recommendations on how one can include sweets into a diabetic-friendly diet plan.

Before doing so, the following are some effective tricks in cutting down sugar in meals:

1. *Reducing the quantity of sodas and juices*

   Science has proven that the risks associated with diabetes increase by 15 percent for every 12 ounce serving of sugar-sweetened drinks. If you are craving a carbonation kick, you can drink sparkling water instead, then add lime, lemon or fruit juice to it. For coffees and teas, you must lessen the amount of sweeteners and creamers.

2. *Do-it-yourself sweetening*

   This is a good way to control the amount of sugar that you will get from the food and drinks you will be consuming. For instance, you can buy plain yogurt, as well as unflavored oatmeal or even unsweetened iced tea, and then just add a small quantity of sweeteners by yourself.

3. *Reducing sugar in recipes*

   If the recipe prescribes putting a cup of sugar in the food, you can reduce the quantity by one-quarter or even half.

Alternatively, you can use cinnamon or vanilla extract to add sweetness.

4. *Discovering healthy ways to meet sweet satisfaction*

   There are creative and fun ways to satisfy cravings for sweetness. You just need to unleash the better options. For instance, if you want a cone of ice cream, you can blend some frozen bananas, instead.

5. *Cut your usual dessert portion by half.*

   If you usually eat two slices of cake before, you can still eat a slice and then replace the other slice with some fruits.

8. *Other practical tips in putting sweets into a diabetic-friendly diet plan.*

   • Do not eat bread together with dessert. Sweets add carbohydrates to a meal. You need to cut other carb-containing food in the same meal.
   • Healthy fats could be added to a dessert.
   • Eat sweets after a meal, instead of taking them alone as a snack.
   • Savour each bite of the dessert you are eating.

Tip #3: Pick the right fats

Fat is a taboo word in a healthy diet. People always see its bad side. This is because fats can either be harmful or helpful. However, our body still needs fat. As is repeatedly stated in this guide, the key here is moderation. In this regard, you need to be smart in choosing the fats that you are going to take. You need to know the fact that fat has both unhealthy and healthy impacts on your body. You just need to unlock its good side to benefit from it. Nevertheless, you need to keep in mind that fats are high in calories too, which means that you need to be watchful of your caloric content.

To accomplish this, you need to make a delineation between healthy and unhealthy fats.

> • *Healthy fats* – these unsaturated fats are found in plants and fish. Primary sources include olive and canola oils, nuts, and avocados. You can focus on omega-3 fatty acids too. These fight inflammation and support a healthy brain and heart. They can be found in salmon, tuna, and flaxseeds.

> • *Unhealthy fats* - as stated in the previous sections, you need to avoid saturated and trans fats because they are damaging kinds of fats. The former kind of fat is commonly found in various animal products like red meat, dairy products and eggs. The latter is common in processed or preserved foods.

Knowing the difference between healthy and unhealthy fats, there are some tips that are very useful in crafting your diet plan. These include the following:

> • Use olive oil, rather than vegetable or butter oil, when cooking.
> • Trim fat from meats before cooking them or remove the skin of the chicken.
> • Try eating nuts or seeds for snacks, instead of chips and crackers.

• You can grill, broil, bake or stir-fry, instead of frying or deep frying.
• You can serve fish at least twice a week, instead of red meat meals.
• If you love cheese, try to replace it with avocado.
• Using canola oil or applesauce in baking is a better option.
• Try adding low-fat milk and flour for a creamier soup, instead of heavy cream.

Chapter 5

Maintaining A Healthy Weight

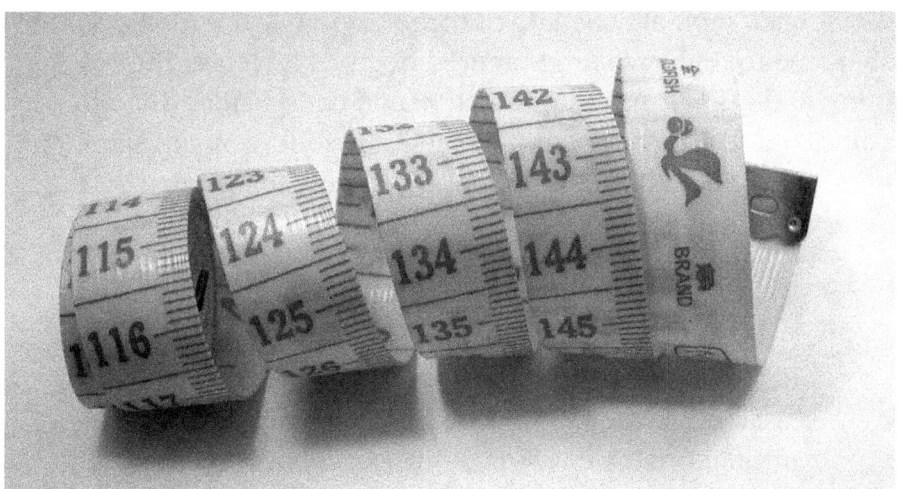

According to some studies, overweight people only need to lose approximately seven percent of their body weight in order to cut in half the risk of developing diabetes. What this means is that overweight people do not have to be obsessive in counting calories or even starving themselves in order to get out of the danger zone.

Aside from that, various research also shows that two (2) of the most powerful and helpful strategies when it comes to weight loss are about regularity and recording. In other words, they are about regularly eating meals according to schedule and recording the kind of food taken.

Eating regularly

On the one hand, there are lots of studies proving that the body is able to regulate blood sugar levels better, when there is a maintained regular schedule of meals. Doing this will also allow someone to regulate weight more effectively. Hence, the best thing to do is to aim for moderation and consistency when it comes to the time and size of meals. The following are some helpful tips that you should know to execute this strategy:

• *Never skip breakfast*

Breakfast marks the start of the day. It provides energy that one needs for the entire day. Also, not skipping breakfast will let you have stable blood sugar levels throughout the day. In contrast, skipping breakfast will make you want to eat more in the latter part of the day, which will shoot up your blood sugar level.

• *Eat small, but up to six meals in a day*

If you think that eating less frequently makes you lose weight faster, then you are wrong. This is because it is alright to eat even up to six times a day, as long as the serving size is small. This is much better than having few, but bigger in size, meals.

• *Keep the same calorie intake*

Regulating the amount of calories you are consuming daily will always be an important part of a healthy diet. This is because it has an impact on blood sugar levels.

Food Diary

People who keep a food diary are likely to be successful in losing weight and maintaining that weight loss. According to some studies, people like these are inclined to lose twice as much weight than people who are not keeping a food diary. This is because tracking food consumed makes a person conscious of the kinds of food he or she is eating. One is reminded of the things to do, success, and progress with respect to the diet plan.

A food diary can be used too in tracking and monitoring success of the diet plan, with respect to expectations. The following table can be adopted in doing this:

Table 5. Sample expectation table

Expectation 1	Blood sugar level at the end of: 1st week : 2nd week : 3rd week : 4th week (end of month) :
Expectation 2	
Expectation 3	
Expectation 4	
Expectation 4	

Engaging in physical activities

Increasing engagement in physical activities is helpful in controlling your blood sugar level. This is because you are burning some excess fat from the food you eat, which will only turn into sugar in your blood if you do not exercise.

Having a carb-protein-fat guideline

The following table provides a simple guide on how much carbohydrates, protein and vegetables a regular person should take in a day, with three full meals and three snacks.

Table 6.
Daily carbohydrates, protein and vegetables consumption

Time	Carbohydrates	Protein	Vegetable or fat
Breakfast	2 to 3 choices (30 to 45 grams)	Meat, poultry, fish, eggs, cheese and peanut butter	Freely
Morning snack	1 to 2 choices (15 to 30 grams)	Same as above	Freely
Lunch	3 to 4 choices (45 to 60 grams)	Same as above	Freely
Afternoon snack	1 to 2 choices (15 to 30	Same as above	Freely

	grams)		
Dinner	3 to 4 choices (45 to 60 grams)	Same as above	Freely
Evening snack	1 to 2 choices (15 to 30 grams)	Same as above	Freely

Chapter 6

How To Motivate Yourself To Manage Your Diabetes

Two of the main reasons why people cannot sustain their healthy diet plan are lack of rules and preparing boring food. Lack of rules is about not having the list of dos and don'ts while having boring food is about absence of creativity. As stated above, it is not true that the food that diabetic people should eat is sweet-less. Healthy food should not be tasteless. With that, the following can be followed:

Setting rules

Without formulating these, there is a high chance that you will just fail following your supposedly healthy diet and not control or manage your blood sugar level at all. Discipline is always the key to successfully managing your blood sugar level. Though this may sound simple, it would be a continuous struggle. You need to keep in mind that you MUST obey your rules in order to achieve your EXPECTATION, which is to control your blood sugar level and become healthier.

The following are some of the do's and don'ts that can be followed:

DO'S:
- Follow your rules!
- Set a goal or target. This could be about the blood sugar level that you want to achieve at the end of the week or month.
- Create a month-long diet meal calendar.

- Include meals that will excite you. You must be creative here!
- Innovate and reinvent meals for purposes of having a variety of meals without compromising its nutritional content.
- Kill monotony and boredom! You don't have to eat tasteless meals every single day. You can set themes or motifs for a day. For example, it can be high-fibre on Mondays while protein-rich on Tuesdays and so on.

DON'TS:

- Break your own rules!
- Get demoralized or demotivated.
- Have a "there's medicine, anyway" mindset.

Creative and fun meals

Trying the following recipes adds fun and colour to the table. The best part here is that they are not difficult to prepare at all.

Table 7. Suggested Recipes, per time of serving

Suggested Time of Serving	Recipe
Brunch or lunch	Spanish Style Arroz con Pollo With Rice
Lunch or dinner	Beef Pozole
Snack or breakfast	Tropical Fruits Fantasia (Fanstasia de Frutas Tropicales

The ingredients and directions in preparing these recipes can be searched on the internet. For specific creative recipes, the following are also recommended:

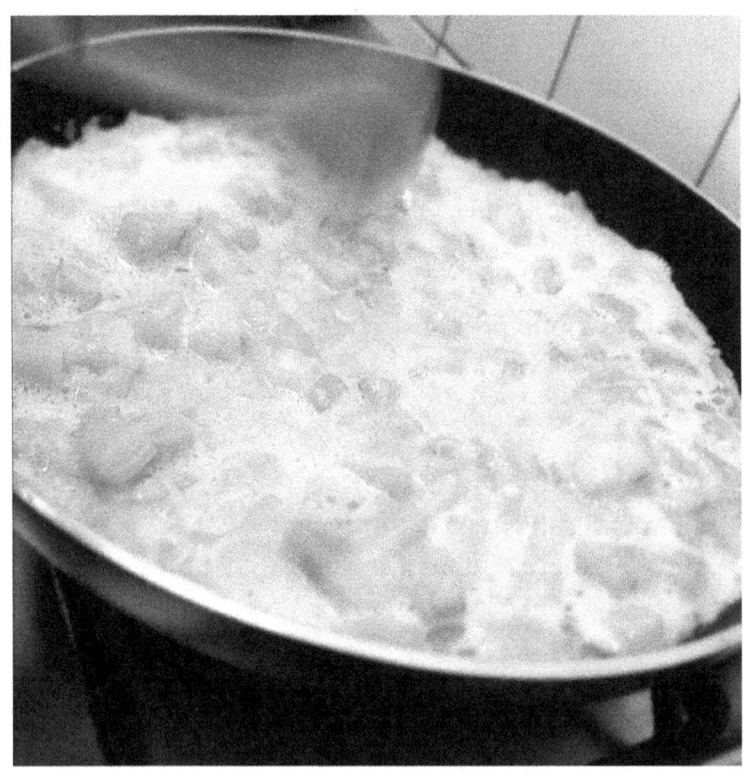

Breakfast: Spanish Omelette (Tortilla Espanola)

The Spanish Omelette or Tortilla Espanola is a tasty dish to start your day. You can have it as a snack too. If you want to serve it for lunch or dinner, it would be best to match it with fresh fruit salad or a whole-grain dinner roll. This dish is packed with the health benefits of the vegetables in it.

Table 8.
Ingredients and directions in preparing Spanish Omelette

Ingredients	Directions
• **5 pieces of small potatoes (peeled and sliced)** • **Vegetable cooking spray** • **½ medium-sized onion (minced)** • **1 small zucchini (sliced)** • **1 ½ cups of green or red bell peppers (sliced thinly)** • **5 medium-sized mushrooms (sliced)** • **3 whole eggs (beaten)** • **5 egg whites (beaten)** • **Pepper and garlic salt**	1. Preheat the oven to 375 degrees Fahrenheit. 2. Boil water and cook the potatoes there until they are tender. 3. Add vegetable spray to a non-stick pan until it is warm to medium heat. 4. Sauté the onions in the non-stick pan until brown. 5. Add vegetables and sauté until half-cooked. 6. Mix the beaten whole eggs and egg whites together with pepper, garlic salt and mozzarella cheese. After mixing, stir the mixture into the half-cooked vegetables. 7. Using an ovenproof skillet or pie pan, add vegetable spray and then transfer the potatoes to the pan, together with the egg-cheese mixture. 8. Sprinkle with low-fat parmesan cheese. 9. Bake for around 20 to 30 minutes or until its texture is firm and its top is brown. 10. Once cooked, remove the omelette from the oven and let cool for 10 minutes. 11. Cut the Spanish Omelette into five (5) slices or in the preferred serving size.

- **(with herbs)**
- **3 ounces of shredded mozzarella cheese**
- **1 tablespoon of low-fat parmesan cheese**

Lunch: Beef or Turkey Stew

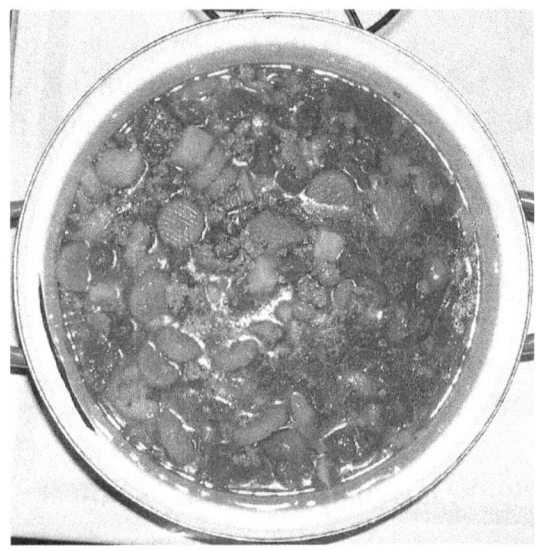

For something heavy and healthy for lunch, one of the options is Beef Stew. You can replace beef with turkey if you want. It goes well with fresh lettuce and cucumber salad on the side or just a dinner roll. Instead of the potatoes, you can use plantains or corn as well.

Table 9.
Ingredients and Directions in Preparing Beef or Turkey Stew

Ingredients	Directions
• **1 pound lean beef (you may also use turkey breast) (cut into cubes)** • **2 tablespoons whole wheat flour** • **¼ teaspoon salt (optional)** • **¼ teaspoon pepper** • **¼ teaspoon cumin** • **1 ½ teaspoon olive oil** • **2 cloves garlic (minced)** • **2 medium-sized onions (sliced)** • **2 stalks celery (sliced)** • **1 medium red or green bell pepper (sliced)** • **1 medium-sized tomato (finely minced)** • **5 cups beef (or turkey) broth (remove the fat)** • **5 pieces small potatoes (peeled and cubed)** • **12 pieces small carrots (cut into**	1. Preheat oven to 375 degrees Fahrenheit. 2. Mix the whole-wheat flour, salt, pepper and cumin. 3. Roll the beef (or turkey) cubes in the mixture. 4. Shake off the excess flour. 5. Heat the olive oil in the skillet in medium to high heat. 6. Once the olive oil is already hot, add the beef (or turkey) cubes. Saute them until nicely brown for around 7 to 10 minutes. 7. Place the sauted beef (or turkey) in your ovenproof casserole dish. 8. Add the garlic, onions, celery and pepper to the skillet. Cook for around 5 minutes or until the vegetables are tender. 9. Add tomato and broth to the skillet, then bring to a boil. 10. Pour over the beef (or turkey) into the casserole dish. 11. Cover tightly, then bake for an hour. 12. Remove disk from the oven and stir in the small potatoes, carrots, and peas. 13. Cook for another 20 to 25 minutes or until its texture is already tender.

chunks)
• 1 ¼ cups green peas

Dinner 1: Caribbean Red Snapper or Pargo Rojo Caribeno

Fish is good for dinner. This can be served with vegetables on top of whole-grain or brown rice. Garnish with parsley for a mouth-watering look. Instead of using red snapper, you can use salmon or chicken breast for something heavier, but healthy, for the tummy.

**Table 10.
Ingredients and Directions in Preparing Caribbean Red Snapper**

Ingredients	Directions
• **2 tablespoons olive oil** • **1 medium-sized onion (chopped)** • **½ cup red bell pepper (chopped)** • **½ cup carrots (cut into strips)** • **1 clove garlic (minced)** • **½ cup dry white wine** • **¾ pound red snapper fillet** • **1 large tomato (chopped)** • **2 tablespoons pitted ripe olives**	1. Heat olive oil in a large skillet over medium heat. 2. Put chopped onion, red bell pepper, carrots and garlic. 3. Saute mixture for 10 minutes. 4. Add white wine and bring to a boil. 5. Push vegetables to the side of the pan. 6. Arrange red snapper fillet in single layer at the centre of the skillet. 7. Cover it and cook for 5 minutes. 8. Add tomato and olives, then top with cheese. 9. Cover skillet and cook for another 3 minutes or until the fish is already firm, but moist. 10. Transfer fish to the serving platter. 11. Garnish plate with vegetables and

(chopped)	pan juices.
• **2 tablespoons crumbled low-fat feta (alternative: low-fat ricotta cheese).**	12.Serve dish with whole-grain or brown rice.

Chapter 7

Three Simple Lifestyle Changes Which Will Help You Cure Your Diabetes

Aside from picking the right kinds of food to eat, there are at least three (3) simple, but high impact, lifestyle changes that will help diabetic people in curing and reversing diabetes. These are, in fact, frequently reiterated in the entire report. They are the following:

1.   *Changing mind set*

There are some people who tend to just embrace the status quo when diagnosed with diabetes. In other words, they just accept that they have it and think that there is nothing that they can do anymore. So, they live life innocently, with the thinking that they are living it to the fullest, but without knowing that they can reverse the condition. Of course, there are already ways to treat diabetes, but such medications will never be sustainably effective without a paradigm shift. First, you need to believe that you can do something about it.

2.   *Having Discipline*

Sticking to a healthy diet plan is a struggle that you need to live every single day. Yes, it is not easy, but it is definitely worth it. Discipline is very vital here, together with determination. For some tips on the do's and don'ts, you may refer to the rules stated in Chapter 6 above.

3.   *Getting active*

Any diet plan is a sure fail in the long run without physical activity. You need to get active in order to have a good physique. This does not mean that you have to go to the gym every day. This could be in simple ways like home-based weight lifting for 30 minutes, jogging, walking and running. The key here is regularity.

Conclusion

This report addressed and provided some enlightenment to people with Type 2 diabetes. Chapter 1 discussed in more depth the characteristics and general description of Type 2 diabetes, as well as its signs or symptoms and even understanding blood sugar levels.

This was followed by reiterating the importance of proper nutrition in Chapter 2, specifically about defining what healthy eating is and deconstructing some myths related to a diabetic diet plan. The concept, uses and applications of Glycemic Index in various food products were also explored in Chapter 3 while Chapter 4 focused on creating your own diet plan in the most affordable way. Some tips and alternatives of the "usual" kinds of food that a diabetic person can eat were given in the said Chapter.

Some tips on how to maintain a healthy weight were discussed in Chapter 5, particularly through keeping a food diary and engaging in physical activities. Chapters 6 and 7 dealt more about inculcating lifestyle changes in order to sustainably prevent, and eventually cure, Type 2 diabetes.

In general, there are at least three (3) lessons that this report discussed, which are:

1. You can do something about Type 2 diabetes, in monitoring, lowering and reversing it.
2. Dieting is partly about the amount of food you eat, but about the kinds of food too.
3. It is not true that you will have a boring "eating" life when you have diabetes. You can still eat sweets, but you just need to be "sweet-smart."

4.   Dieting, aside from regulating the quantity and quality, should include exercise too for it to be effective in the long-run.

REFERENCES:

Diabetes Digital Media Ltd. (n.d.). Blood Sugar Level Ranges.
    [ONLINE] Available at:
    http://www.diabetes.co.uk/diabetes_care/blood-sugar-
    level-ranges.html. [Last Accessed 08 June 2014].

Ludwig, D. and Rostler, S., (2007). Ending the Food Fight: Guide
    Your Child to a Healthy Weight in a Fast Food/Fake Food
    World. United States of America: Houghton Mifflin
    Company.

University of Maryland Medical Center (2012). Diabetes Diet.
    [ONLINE] Available at:
    http://umm.edu/health/medical/reports/articles/diabetes-
    diet. [Last Accessed 08 June 2014].

World Heath Organization (WHO) (2013). Diabetes. [ONLINE]
    Available at:
    http://www.who.int/mediacentre/factsheets/fs312/en/ .
    [Last Accessed 8 June 2014].

World Heath Organization (WHO) Department of
    Noncommunicable Disease Surveillance, (1999).
    Definition, diagnosis and classification of diabetes mellitus
    and its complications. Part 1: Diagnosis and classification
    of diabetes mellitus. Geneva: World Health Organization.

Other Books By Dr Brad Turner

Headache Cures Made Easy

Headaches are extremely common, especially in today's society where everyone is stressed, exhausted and forever taking on too much work. However, the big problem arises when we stop viewing headaches as something serious. Whether large or small, headaches can often be a symptom of a more severe underlying problem and ignoring them is the worst thing we can do. Whether you regularly experience primary or secondary headaches, you can use this guide to learn about the causes of headaches, the symptoms that can arise and how to tackle them if they are a common occurrence in your life. It also offers you details of natural cures, giving you useful tips and ideas to help stop that headache in its tracks, as well as information on how to prevent getting headaches and migraines in the future.

Lose Belly Fat Without Exercise

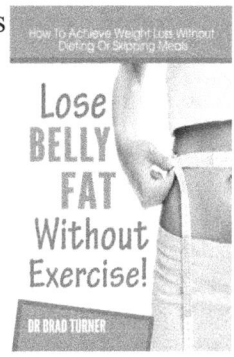

Dr Brad Turner's *Lose Belly Fat Without Exercise* is an easy to follow guide which gives you the important information you need to give you a jump start to a vibrant, radiant and sexy new you!

If you are tired of counting calories, fat grams and points and or have lost your motivation with crash course exercise programs and are tired of diets that just do not work, then this book is for you.

Aromatherapy The Beginner's Guide

Frankincense. Peppermint. Eucalyptus. Lemon-grass. Lavender. Who knew that these are five must-have essential oils? Dr. Brad Turner does—and we are blessed that he's chosen to share his knowledge and expertise in his latest book, ESSENTIAL OILS. So much has been written about using oils: As cures for everything from toothaches to acne; aromatherapy and even taken internally for whatever reason is popular that day.. To our own peril, we've discovered much of this information is false. Dr.

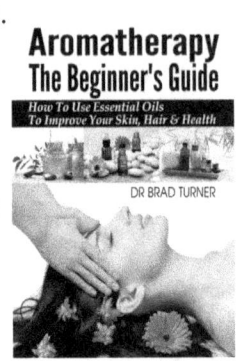

Turner gains our trust immediately with his treatise: Never ingest these essential oils. And that's the beginning of an author/reader relationship that will stand the test of time…and information, because Dr. Turner tells the truth. And that's the way we like it!

Quit Smoking Naturally

On every literary corner, there's an expert on how to quit smoking. But very few of their theories stick. Every day the weary smoker is inspired to quit, only to have his/her hopes dashed yet again.*Quit Smoking Naturally* is the book that may set everyone free! The genius of this book is the straightforward approach and authentic voice that provides the facts, dispels the fallacies and motivates the smoker to do what they've never done before—succeed at quitting!

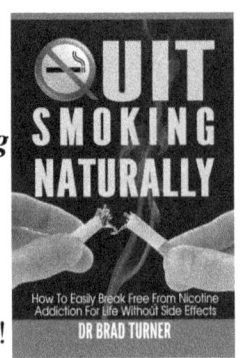

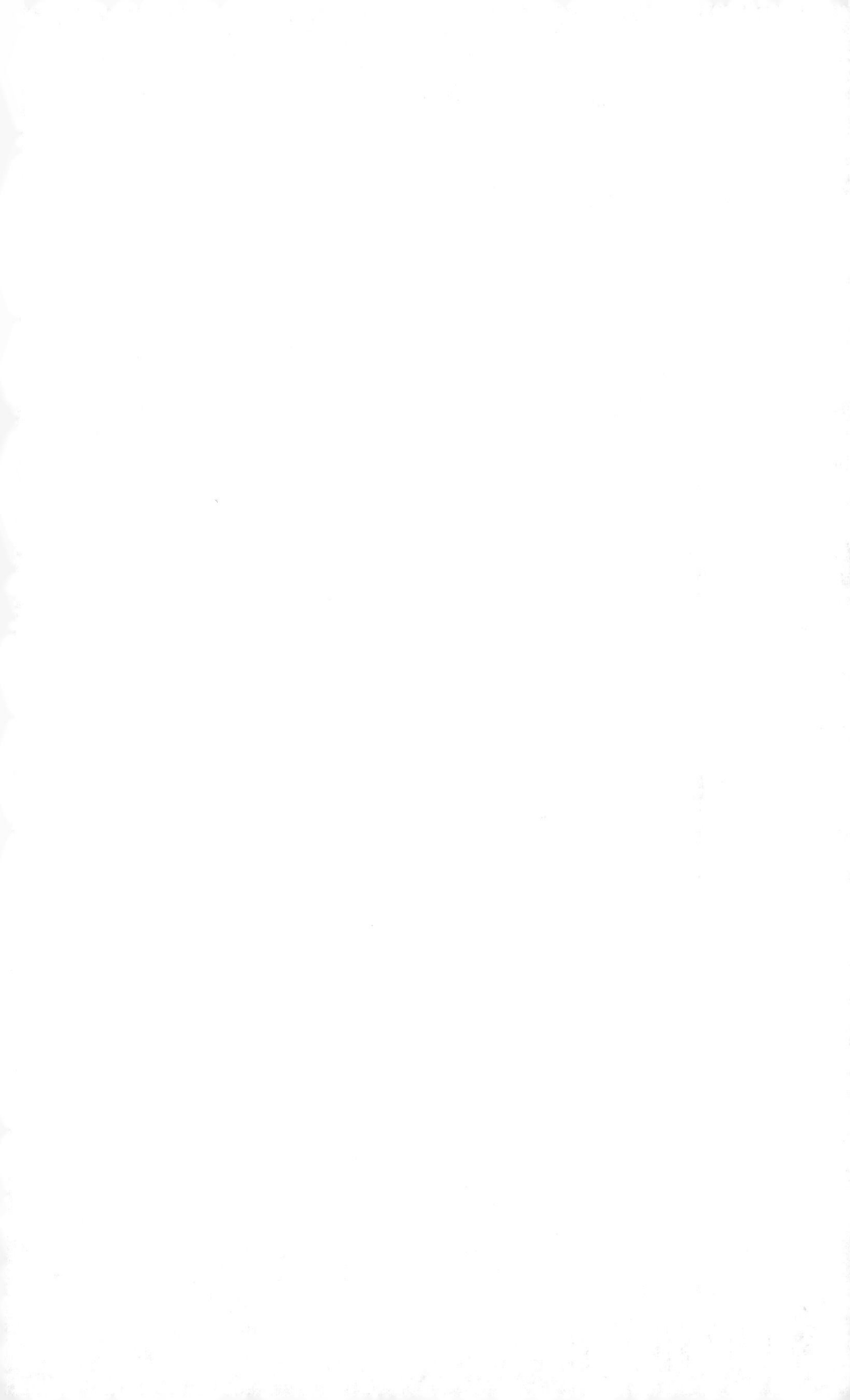

www.ingramcontent.com/pod-product-compliance
Lightning Source LLC
Chambersburg PA
CBHW070233290526
45789CB00004B/1608